Vegan Diet

Vegan Diet for Beginners with Clean Eating and Delicious Easy Recipes for a New Healthy Vegan Lifestyle

Jessie Mills

Published by Robert Satterfield Publishing House

© **Jessie Mills**

All Rights Reserved

Vegan diet: Vegan Diet for Beginners with Clean Eating and Delicious Easy Recipes for a New Healthy Vegan Lifestyle

ISBN 978-1-989682-78-4

All rights reserved. No part of this guide may be reproduced in any form without permission in writing from the publisher except in the case of brief quotations embodied in critical articles or reviews.

Legal & Disclaimer

The information contained in this book is not designed to replace or take the place of any form of medicine or professional medical advice. The information in this book has been provided for educational and entertainment purposes only.

The information contained in this book has been compiled from sources deemed reliable, and it is accurate to the best of the Author's knowledge; however, the Author cannot guarantee its accuracy and validity and cannot be held liable for any errors or omissions. Changes are periodically made to this book. You must consult your doctor or get professional medical advice before using any of the suggested remedies, techniques, or information in this book.

TABLE OF CONTENT

Part 1 1

Introduction... 2

Vegan Vanilla Cupcakes... 3

Orange Cake 5

Moist Vegan Chocolate Cake With Frosting......................... 6

Vegan Apple Spice Cake 8

Chocolate Pudding 10

Vegan Walnut Brownies 11

Vegan Cheesecake... 14

Vegan Chocolate Espresso Ice Cream 15

Zucchini Chocolate Cake.. 17

Carrot Cake.. 19

Pumpkin Pie... 21

Coconut Truffles 22

Pecan Coffee Cake... 24

Brown Sugar Squares 27

Peanut Butter Brownies 28

Creamy Chocolate Vegan Cake.. 30

Lime Sorbet 32

Cherry Crisp 34

Chai Tea Coconut Brownies	35
Apple Pie	37
CRUST	37
Key Lime Pie	41
CRUST	41
FILLING	41
Chocolate Banana Cake	43
Vegan Apple Cheesecake	45
No Bake Strawberry Vegan Cheesecake	47
FILLING	48
TOPPING	48
Dark Chocolate Brownies	50
Zucchini Brownies	53
Vegan Chocolate Cheesecake	54
CRUST	54
Part 2	56
Introduction	58
Chapter 1: Vegan Cake Recipes	59
Pineapple Upside Down Cake	59
Banana Chocolate Cake	61
Chocolate Vegan Cake	62
Spiced Coconut Cake	64

Vegan Fudge Cake 65

Vegan Pumpkin Cheesecake.. 66

FILLING: 67

Chocolate Zucchini Cake.. 68

Pound Cake.. 69

Orange Cake 71

Creamy Tofu Chocolate Cake 72

Chapter 2: Vegan Cookie Recipes...................................... 75

Snickerdoodle Cookies 75

Gingersnap Cookies... 76

Vegan Oatmeal Cookies 78

Chia Seed Cookies 80

Moist Lemon Cookies 82

Chocolate Oatmeal Cookies 83

Banana Oatmeal Cookies 84

Vegan Butter Cookies.. 86

Sugar Cookies 88

Chocolate Fudge Cookies 90

Peanut Butter Cookies... 91

Chapter 3: Vegan Muffin Recipes...................................... 93

Banana Muffins 93

Oat Muffins 94

Cornbread Muffins	96
Apple Carrot Muffins	98
Pumpkin Muffins	99
Classic Zucchini Muffins	101
Pecan Muffins	103
Bran Muffins	105
About The Author	108

Part 1

Introduction

There are many great reasons to try the vegan diet! One reason why many people choose to go on this diet is because it is because you will not be consuming any dairy products which contain animal hormones and fats. It is known that consuming dairy and meats can cause health problems like obesity, cancer and heart disease. The vegan diet is healthy because you will not be consuming high amounts of fat, and carcinogens that meat has been shown to contain.

When I first started the vegan diet years ago, I immediately noticed my health improve, along with my mood and quality of life. It is unfortunate that many people will not experience the benefits of the vegan diet, but it is my hope that these vegan recipes will help convert non-vegans!

This vegan dessert cookbook includes tasty vegan dessert recipes that range from cookies, cakes and brownies. All of these dessert recipes are dairy and egg free. Good luck and we hope you enjoy this vegan dessert cookbook.

Vegan Vanilla Cupcakes

Makes 12-14 cupcakes

Ingredients

½ cup plain coconut milk

1 cup warm water

3 tablespoon grapeseed oil

1 tablespoon vanilla

1 teaspoon lemon juice

¼ cup unsweetened applesauce

¾ cup organic brown rice flour

¾ cup tapioca flour

½ cup organic coconut flour

1 cup organic cane sugar

½ teaspoon sea salt

1 teaspoon baking powder

1 teaspoon baking soda

1 teaspoon xanthan gum

Directions

Preheat oven to 375F.

Measure the non-dairy milk into a liquid measuring cup and add lemon juice. Set aside.

Whisk together all dry ingredients.

Add all liquid ingredients to the dry ingredients and mix with electric mixer until smooth.

Fill the cupcake wrappers with mixture.

Bake for 15-20 minutes. Cupcakes will be golden brown when done.

Orange Cake

Ingredients

1 1/2 cups all-purpose flour

1 large orange, peeled

1 cup white sugar

1/2 cup vegetable oil

1 1/2 teaspoons baking soda

1/4 teaspoon salt

Directions

Preheat oven to 375F. Grease an 8x8-inch baking pan.

Blend orange in the blender until liquified; measure 1 cup orange juice.

Whisk orange juice, flour, sugar, vegetable oil, baking soda, and salt together in a bowl. Pour batter into the prepared pan.

Bake in the preheated oven until a toothpick inserted in the center of the cake comes out clean, about 30 minutes.

Moist Vegan Chocolate Cake With Frosting

Ingredients
1 ¼ cup all-purpose flour
1 cup sugar
⅓ cup cocoa powder

1 teaspoon baking soda

½ teaspoon salt

1 cup warm water

1 teaspoon vanilla extract

⅓ cup vegetable oil

1 teaspoon white or apple cider vinegar

For frosting

½ cup sugar

4 tablespoons margarine or vegan butter substitute

2 tablespoons soy milk

2 tablespoons cocoa powder

2 teaspoons vanilla extract

Directions

Preheat oven to 350F.

In an 8 x 8 inch square pan, mix the flour, sugar, cocoa powder, baking soda and salt with a fork. Add the water, vanilla extract, vegetable oil and vinegar.

Mix the ingredients together. Bake for 30 minutes. Cool on a cooling rack.

To Make Frosting:
In a small saucepan bring the sugar, margarine, soy milk and cocoa powder to a boil, stirring frequently.

Simmer for 2 minutes, remove from heat and stir an additional 5 minutes. Stir in the vanilla extract.

Pour the glaze onto cake and let it cool for one hour.

Vegan Apple Spice Cake

Ingredients

¾ cup apple sauce

½ cup sugar

1 teaspoons vanilla extract

½ teaspoon salt

½ teaspoon cinnamon

¼ teaspoon nutmeg

¼ teaspoon allspice

1 tablespoon brown rice syrup

6 tablespoons non-dairy milk

1 teaspoon apple cider vinegar

1 ¼ cup all purpose flour

1 ½ teaspoon non-aluminum baking powder

½ teaspoon baking soda

Directions

Preheat oven to 350F.

In a medium size bowl, whisk non-dairy milk the with apple cider vinegar and set aside for 5 to 10 minutes so it lightly curdles.

In a medium size mixing bowl whisk together the all purpose flour, baking powder, baking soda and set aside.

In a large mixing bowl, mix the apple sauce, sugar, vanilla extract, salt, cinnamon, nutmeg, allspice, brown rice syrup and the non-dairy milk apple cider mixture.

Add the flour mixture to the mixing bowl containing the wet ingredients and mix until combined.

Pour mixture into an oiled 8 inch round cake pan and bake for about 25 minutes or until an inserted toothpick comes out clean.

Chocolate Pudding

Ingredients

2 large avocados - peeled, pitted, and cubed

1/2 cup unsweetened cocoa powder

1/2 cup brown sugar

1/3 cup coconut milk

2 teaspoons vanilla extract

1 pinch ground cinnamon

Directions

Blend avocados, cocoa powder, brown sugar, coconut milk, vanilla extract, and cinnamon in a blender until smooth.

Refrigerate pudding until chilled, about 30 minutes.

Vegan Walnut Brownies

Ingredients

1 ¾ cups all-purpose flour

¼ teaspoon baking soda

7 tablespoons cocoa powder

4 ounces semi-sweet chocolate, chopped into ¼ inch pieces

1 teaspoon instant espresso powder

¾ teaspoon salt

¼ cup boiling water

1 ½ cups sugar

6 tablespoons non-hydrogenated stick margarine, melted

1 ½ teaspoons vanilla extract

½ cup walnuts, chopped

Directions

In a small mixing bowl whisk together the water and flax meal. Let it sit for about 10 minutes so the mixture thickens. Ensure oven rack is in the middle rack position.

Preheat your oven to 350F.

Line an 8 x 8 inch baking dish with parchment paper, allow excess parchment paper on opposite sides to remove brownies easier from baking dish when finished baking.

In a medium mixing bowl whisk together the all-purpose flour and baking soda. Set aside.

In another medium mixing bowl add the cocoa powder, semi-sweet chocolate, espresso powder and salt. Add the boiling water and using a spoon, mix in the ingredients into a paste, making sure that all of the chocolate pieces are melted.

Add the sugar, margarine, vanilla extract, flax meal mixture from the first step into the chocolate mixture and mix with an electric mixer until smooth.

Stir in the walnuts and mix in the flour with a spoon until well combined. Use your hands to mix, since the mixture will be very thick. Do not use an electric mixer for mixing.

Transfer the batter to the baking dish. You may need to use your fingers or a spatula to press the thick dough into place.

Bake for 25 minutes on the middle rack in the oven. Transfer the baking dish to a wire cooling rack and allow it to cool for about an hour.

Cool completely before slicing.

Vegan Cheesecake

Ingredients
1 (12 ounce) package soft tofu
1/2 cup soy milk
1/2 cup white sugar

1 tablespoon vanilla extract

1/4 cup maple syrup

1 (9 inch) prepared graham cracker crust

Directions

Preheat oven to 350F.

In a blender, combine the tofu, soy milk, sugar, vanilla extract and maple syrup. Blend until smooth and pour into pie crust.

Bake at 350F for 30 minutes. Remove from oven, allow to cool and refrigerate until chilled.

Vegan Chocolate Espresso Ice Cream

Ingredients

1/2 (12 ounce) package extra-firm silken tofu

1 cup soy milk

1 tablespoon hazelnut flavored syrup

4 teaspoons instant espresso powder

1 teaspoon vanilla extract

2/3 cup semisweet vegan chocolate chips, melted

Directions

Place the tofu, soy milk, hazelnut syrup, espresso powder, and vanilla extract into a blender.

Cover, and puree until smooth. Pour in the melted chocolate, and puree until evenly incorporated. Pour the mixture into a bowl, cover, and refrigerate until cold, at least 1 hour.

Pour the chilled mixture into an ice cream maker and freeze according to the manufacturer's directions. Once the ice cream has thickened and is hard to stir, remove it from the ice cream maker and transfer it to a freezer container.

Allow the ice cream to harden 4 hours to overnight before serving.

Zucchini Chocolate Cake

Ingredients

2 cups flour

1 ¾ cups raw sugar

¾ cup cocoa powder

¾ cup chickpea flour

1 teaspoon baking soda

½ teaspoon baking powder

pinch of salt

¾ cup oil or apple purée

¾ cup water

1 ½– 2 cups grated zucchini

2 teaspoons vanilla extract

Directions

Preheat the oven to 375F.

Grease and flour a large bundt pan.

In a mixing bowl combine the flour, sugar, cocoa, chickpea flour, baking soda, baking powder and salt. Break up any lumps and mix until evenly combined.

In a separate mixing bowl combine the oil, water, zucchini and vanilla. Add this mixture to the dry ingredients, stirring until no traces of flour remain.

Pour into the bundt tin and bake for 1 hour, until the top is firm and a toothpick comes out clean.

Let cool for 10 minutes before removing from pan.

Carrot Cake

Ingredients

2 cups whole wheat flour

1/4 cup soy flour (optional)

1 1/2 tablespoons ground cinnamon

1 tablespoon ground cloves

4 teaspoons baking soda

2 teaspoons tapioca starch (optional)

1/2 teaspoon salt

1 1/2 cups hot water

1/4 cup flax seed meal

2 cups packed brown sugar

4 teaspoons vanilla extract

3/4 cup dried currants (optional)

6 carrots, grated

1/2 cup blanched slivered almonds

Directions

Preheat oven to 350F.

Prepare a 9x13 inch baking pan with cooking spray. Whisk together the whole wheat flour, soy flour, cinnamon, ground cloves, baking soda, tapioca starch, and salt in a bowl until blended; set aside.

Pour the hot water into a mixing bowl, and sprinkle with the flax meal. Stir for a minute until the flax begins to absorb the water, and the mixture slightly thickens.

Stir in the brown sugar and vanilla until the sugar has dissolved, then add the currants, carrots, and almonds. Stir in the dry mixture until just moistened, then pour into the prepared pan.

Bake in the preheated oven until a toothpick inserted into the center comes out clean, about 30 minutes.

Cool in the pan for 10 minutes before removing to cool completely on a wire rack.

Pumpkin Pie

Ingredients

1 (10.5 ounce) package silken tofu, drained

1 (16 ounce) can pumpkin puree

3/4 cup white sugar

1/2 teaspoon salt

1 teaspoon ground cinnamon

1/2 teaspoon ground ginger

1/4 teaspoon ground cloves

1 (9 inch) unbaked pie crust

Directions

Preheat an oven to 450F.

Place the tofu, pumpkin, sugar, salt, cinnamon, ginger, and clove into a blender. Puree until smooth. Pour into the pie crust.

Bake in the preheated oven 15 minutes, then reduce heat to 350F, and continue baking until a knife inserted into the mixture comes out clean, about 40 minutes more.

Cool before serving.

Coconut Truffles

Ingredients

1 1/4 cups shredded unsweetened coconut, or to taste, divided

2 cups pitted Medjool dates

1 cup raw almonds

2 1/4 cups raw cocoa powder

1/2 cup cocoa nibs

1/2 cup agave nectar

2 teaspoons vanilla extract

1 teaspoon salt

Directions

Preheat oven to 350F. Spread coconut out on a baking sheet. Line a separate baking sheet with parchment paper.

Bake coconut in the preheated oven, stirring occasionally, until golden and toasted, about 7 minutes.

Blend dates and almonds together in a food processor until smooth; add cocoa powder and process until completely incorporated. Transfer date mixture to a bowl.

Fold 1 cup toasted coconut, cocoa nibs, agave nectar, vanilla extract, and salt into date mixture until truffle dough is evenly mixed. Roll dough into tablespoon-size balls.

Pour remaining toasted coconut into a shallow bowl. Roll truffle balls in toasted coconut to coat; place coated truffles on the parchment-lined baking sheet.

Refrigerate truffles until hardened, about 1 hour.

Pecan Coffee Cake

Ingredients

1 cup all purpose flour

1 cup whole wheat flour

¼ teaspoon salt

1 teaspoon baking powder

1 cup margarine, softened

1 cup non-dairy yogurt

1 cup sugar

4 ½ tablespoons arrowroot or tapioca flour

2 teaspoons vanilla extract

¾ cup sugar

1 cup granny smith apple, peeled, cored and chopped into ¼ inch size pieces

1 ½ cup chopped pecans

¾ teaspoon ground cinnamon

½ teaspoon allspice

2 tablespoons margarine, melted

Directions

Preheat oven to 350F.

Lightly grease a 9 x 13 inch baking dish with vegetable oil or cooking spray.

In a medium bowl, mix together the sugar, apple pieces, pecans, cinnamon, allspice and melted margarine until crumbly. Set aside.

In a large bowl, whisk together the all purpose flour, whole wheat flour, salt, baking powder and set aside.

In another large bowl, cream the soft margarine until light and fluffy. Gradually beat in non-dairy yogurt, and then beat in the sugar, followed by beating in the arrowroot or tapioca flour.

Stir in the vanilla. By hand, fold in the flour mixture, mixing until just incorporated. Spread half of the batter into the baking pan then top with half of the apple pecan topping.

Spread the other half of the batter into the pan, followed by the other half of the apple pecan topping.

Bake for 35 minutes, or until a toothpick inserted into the center of the cake comes out clean. Wait until cake is completely cooled before removing from the pan.

Brown Sugar Squares

Ingredients

2/3 cup unbleached all-purpose flour

2/3 cup packed brown sugar

1/4 cup finely chopped walnuts

1 teaspoon ground cinnamon

1/4 teaspoon ground cardamom

1/4 teaspoon salt

1/2 teaspoon baking powder

1 cup dates, pitted and chopped

2 eggs equivalent of vegan egg substitute

Directions

Preheat oven to 350F. Lightly oil an 8-inch square baking pan.

Combine flour, brown sugar, chopped walnuts, cinnamon, cardamom, salt, baking powder, and dates; mix well.

Add egg substitute and stir until dry ingredients are moistened.

Spoon batter into prepared pan and bake in preheated oven until toothpick inserted into center comes out clean, about 25 minutes.

Let cool before cutting.

Peanut Butter Brownies

Ingredients

1 cup natural creamy peanut butter

1 (12 ounce) bag vegan chocolate chips

1 1/2 cups white sugar

1 avocado, peeled and pitted

1/2 cup soy milk

1/2 cup canola oil

1 cup whole-wheat flour

1 teaspoon baking powder

1 teaspoon salt

Directions

Preheat oven to 350 degrees F (175 degrees C). Grease a 9x13-inch baking pan.

Melt peanut butter, chocolate chips, and sugar together in a saucepan over low heat, stirring constantly, until chocolate is melted, about 5 minutes. Increase heat to medium and continue stirring until mixture begins to bubble, about 5 more minutes. Remove from heat.

Blend avocado, soy milk, and canola oil in a food processor until smooth. Stir avocado mixture into chocolate mixture until thoroughly combined.

Whisk flour, baking powder, and salt together in a large bowl until well mixed. Add avocado-chocolate mixture to the flour mixture; stir until just combined. Evenly pour batter into the prepared baking pan.

Bake in the preheated oven until the edges begin to become crisp, for 20 minutes.

Cool brownies completely before cutting and serving.

Creamy Chocolate Vegan Cake

Ingredients

3/4 cup all-purpose flour

1 1/4 cups ground almonds

3/4 cup packed brown sugar, divided

1/2 cup butter

1 1/2 pounds tofu

2/3 cup vegetable oil

1/2 cup orange juice

1/2 cup chocolate liqueur

1/2 cup unsweetened cocoa powder

1 teaspoon almond extract

Directions

Preheat the oven to 325F. Lightly grease a 9 inch springform pan.

In a medium bowl, mix together the flour, ground almonds and 1 tablespoon of the brown sugar. Knead in the butter to form a dough. Press the dough firmly into the bottom of the prepared pan.

Combine the tofu, remaining sugar, oil, orange juice, chocolate liqueur, cocoa, and almond extract using a blender and blend until smooth and creamy. Spread the batter in an even layer over the prepared crust.

Bake for 1 hour and 15 minutes in the preheated oven. Allow cake to cool to room temperature, then refrigerate overnight.

Lime Sorbet

Ingredients
1 cup sugar
1½ cups water

3 pounds ripe mangoes, (3 large or 4 medium), peeled and cut into chunks

¼ cup lime juice

Directions

Combine sugar and water in a saucepan. Stir over medium heat until the liquid comes to a full boil and the sugar has dissolved.

Remove from the heat and let cool to room temperature. Cover with plastic wrap and refrigerate until chilled, about 1 hour.

Puree mango in a food processor or blender. Work the puree through a fine sieve. Measure out 2 cups of and stir into the syrup, along with lime juice.

Freeze the mixture in an ice cream maker according to manufacturer's directions

Serve immediately.

Cherry Crisp

Ingredients

1 (21 ounce) can cherry pie filling

1/2 cup all-purpose flour

1/2 cup rolled oats

2/3 cup brown sugar

3/4 teaspoon ground cinnamon

3/4 teaspoon ground nutmeg

1/4 cup chopped pecans

1/3 cup melted margarine

Directions

Preheat oven to 350F.

Lightly grease a 2 quart baking dish. Pour pie filling into the dish, and spread evenly.

In a medium bowl, mix together flour, oats, sugar, cinnamon, and nutmeg. Mix in melted margarine. Spread over pie filling, and sprinkle with chopped pecans.

Bake in the preheated oven for 30 minutes, or until topping is golden brown.

Allow to cool 15 minutes before serving.

Chai Tea Coconut Brownies

Ingredients

2 tablespoons unsweetened cocoa powder

1 oz unsweetened desiccated coconut

1/2 cup plain flour

7 oz caster sugar

4 tablespoons unsweetened cocoa powder

1/2 teaspoon baking powder

1/2 teaspoon salt

4 fl oz very strongly brewed chai tea

4 fl oz rapeseed oil

1/2 teaspoon vanilla extract

Directions

Preheat an oven to 350F. Spray a square baking pan with cooking spray and dust lightly with the 2 tablespoons cocoa powder.

Place the coconut in the bowl of a food processor, pulse until finely chopped; set aside.

Whisk together the flour, sugar, 4 tablespoons cocoa powder, baking powder and salt.

Stir in the brewed chai, rapeseed oil and vanilla extract, just until all ingredients are moistened.

Fold in the coconut. Spread the batter in the prepared pan.

Bake in the preheated oven until the top is no longer shiny, about 20 minutes. Allow to cool for 1 hour before cutting.

Apple Pie

Ingredients

Crust

1 cup plus 2 tablespoons all-purpose flour

¼ teaspoon salt

6 tablespoons vegan shortening, cut into small pieces

3-4 tablespoons ice water

Filling

8 cups thinly sliced peeled Granny Smith apples

½ cup packed light brown sugar

1 tablespoon lemon juice

½ teaspoon ground cinnamon

1 tablespoon cornstarch

Topping

½ cup rolled oats

¼ cup all-purpose flour

3 tablespoons packed light brown sugar

½ teaspoon ground cinnamon

2 tablespoons vegan shortening

Directions

To Make Crust:

Combine 1 cup plus 2 tablespoons flour and the salt in a large bowl or food processor. Cut in cold shortening using a pastry blender, two knives or by pulsing in the food processor until pebble-size pieces form.

Add ice water, 1 tablespoon at a time, until the dough is evenly moist but not wet and is starting to stick together.

Pat the dough into a 5-inch disk. Lightly flour a large sheet of plastic wrap, place the dough in the center and wrap it up.

Refrigerate for at least 1 hour and or up to 2 days. Remove from the refrigerator about 15 minutes before beginning pie recipe and rolling out.

To Make Filling:

In a large bowl combine apples, ½ cup brown sugar, lemon juice and ½ teaspoon cinnamon. Let mixture stand for at least 10 minutes. Add cornstarch and toss to coat.

Preheat oven to 375°F.

Roll the dough into a 12-inch round between two pieces of parchment paper. Remove the top sheet; gently invert the dough into a 9-inch pie pan.

Remove the second sheet of parchment. Trim the dough to an even overhang all the way around. Patch any cracks with the extra dough. Fold the dough under to form a double layer of crust around the edge. Crimp the edges. Mound the filling into the crust. Bake the pie for 20 minutes.

Prepare Topping:

Combine oats, flour, brown sugar and cinnamon in a medium bowl. Cut in shortening with a pastry blender.

Sprinkle the topping over the pie and continue baking for 40 more minutes until the filling is bubbling and the crust and topping are golden.

Let cool for 1 hour before serving.

Key Lime Pie

Ingredients

Crust
1 cup almond flour
1 cup pitted Medjool dates
1 tablespoon agave nectar
1 teaspoon vanilla extract
1/2 teaspoon salt
1/8 teaspoon ground nutmeg

Filling
5 avocados, peeled and pitted
1/2 cup melted coconut oil
6 tablespoons lime juice

1/4 cup agave nectar

Directions

Blend almond flour, dates, 1 tablespoon agave, vanilla extract, salt, and nutmeg in a food processor until crust sticks together when pinched. Press crust evenly into the bottom of a springform pan.

Process avocados, coconut oil, lime juice, and 1/4 cup agave nectar in a food processor until filling is very smooth; pour over the crust, smoothing with the back of a spoon or spatula.

Freeze pie until set, for at least 4 hours.

Let sit at room temperature for 10 minutes before serving.

Chocolate Banana Cake

Ingredients

3 cups whole wheat pastry flour

3/4 cup white sugar

1/2 cup brown sugar

3/4 cup cocoa powder

2 teaspoons baking powder

1 teaspoon baking soda

1 teaspoon salt

2 cups mashed very ripe bananas

1/2 cup creamy peanut butter

1 1/4 cups almond milk

3/4 cup canola oil

1 (10 ounce) bag semisweet vegan chocolate chips

Directions

Preheat oven to 350F.

Lightly grease a 9x12-inch baking pan.

Mix pastry flour, white sugar, brown sugar, cocoa powder, baking powder, baking soda, and salt together in a bowl. Stir bananas and peanut butter together in a separate bowl until smooth; add almond milk and oil and mix well.

Carefully fold banana mixture into flour mixture until batter is just combined; fold in chocolate chips. Pour batter into the prepared pan.

Bake in the preheated oven until a toothpick inserted in the center comes out clean, 40 to 45 minutes.

Vegan Apple Cheesecake

Ingredients

Vegan graham cracker pie crust

2 ½ cups plain, unsweetened soy yogurt

2 cups almond flour

½ cup non-dairy milk

1 cup sugar

2 Tablespoons unrefined coconut oil

1 Tablespoon + 1 teaspoon lemon juice

2 teaspoons vanilla extract

1 teaspoon salt

2 ½ cups Granny Smith apples, chopped into ¼ inch cubes

2 tablespoons sugar

2 teaspoons unrefined coconut oil

1 ½ teaspoons cinnamon

½ teaspoon nutmeg

½ teaspoon allspice

1 pinch salt

½ cup all-purpose flour or rice flour

Directions

Prepare graham cracker crust in springform pan.

Place the soy yogurt, almond flour and non-dairy milk in a blender and blend for 2 minutes on the highest setting. Transfer the mixture to a bowl.

Preheat oven to 300F.

Transfer the mixture back to the blender and add the sugar, coconut oil, lemon juice, vanilla extract and salt.

Blend for 2 more minutes on the highest setting or until completely smooth.

In a medium frying pan or skillet, add the apples, sugar, coconut oil, cinnamon, nutmeg, allspice and salt. Sauté on medium heat for 10 minutes. Set aside.

Add 1 ¼ cups of the apple mixture to a medium mixing bowl and set aside.

Whisk the ½ cup of all-purpose flour or rice flour into the cheesecake mixture until well combined. Now fold in the apple mixture until barely combined.

Pour the mixture into your prepared spring form pan with crust and bake for 3 hours or until the cheesecake is firm.

Allow the cheesecake to cool completely then transfer it to the refrigerator for a few hours before slicing and serving.

No Bake Strawberry Vegan Cheesecake

Ingredients

1 cup macadamia nuts

1/2 cup walnuts

1/2 cup pitted dates

1/4 cup shredded coconut

Pinch of Himalayan pink salt

Filling

3 cups raw cashews (soaked for 2-4 hours and then drained)

3/4 cup lemon juice

3/4 to 1 cup coconut nectar

3/4 cup coconut oil

1 vanilla bean, split and scraped

Topping

2 cups frozen strawberries

1/2 cup pitted dates

1 cup sliced fresh strawberries, plus 1 cup whole strawberries, to serve

Directions

Lightly grease a round springform pan with coconut oil and line base and sides with baking paper.

Place all ingredients for the crust except for the dates in a food processor, and process until you get the texture of crumbs.

Add dates and process until well combined. Press into the base of the spring form pan and place in the freezer while preparing rest of cheesecake.

In a blender, blend all the ingredients for the filling at high speed until smooth. Pour into the crust layer and return to the freezer until set enough to pour strawberry topping on top.

Clean the blender and blend the frozen strawberries and dates on high speed until smooth.

Pour on top of the cheesecake layer and return to the freezer for 4 hours or overnight.

To serve, remove from freezer and let it sit for 15 minutes at room temperature.

Arrange sliced strawberries on top to serve.

Dark Chocolate Brownies

Ingredients

1 (15.5-ounce) can black beans, drained and rinsed

2 cups water

1/2 cup prunes

1/4 cup packed dark brown sugar

1 teaspoon vanilla extract

1/3 cup dark cocoa powder

1/2 cup oats

1 1/2 cups whole wheat flour

1/2 tsp salt

1 1/2 tsp baking powder

1/2 cup vegan dark chocolate chips

Directions

Preheat the oven to 350°F.

Place the prunes in the bowl of a food processor and pulse a few times until broken down.

Add the black beans and process until smooth, adding a cup of the water in a steady stream to thin the mixture. The beans and prunes should be a smooth texture with a few chunks.

Add the brown sugar and vanilla extract and pulse a few times to combine.

Add the oats, flour, salt and baking powder to the food processor and pulse until combined.

Add the remaining cup of water in a stream until a thick but smooth batter has formed.

Add the chocolate chips and pulse a few times to mix in.

Coat a 9x13-inch baking dish with nonstick cooking spray, then pour in the brownie batter.

Bake 30 minutes, or until a toothpick inserted in the center comes out clean.

Allow to cool before slicing into 12 brownies.

Zucchini Brownies

Ingredients

2 cups grated zucchini

2 tsp vanilla

2 cups whole wheat or whole grain flour

1 tsp salt

1/2 cup light olive oil

1 and 1/4 cup maple syrup

1/4 cup cocoa

1/4 tsp baking soda

Directions

Preheat oven to 350F. Grease and flour a 9 x 13 inch baking pan.

Whisk together the dry ingredients in a bowl. Then add the wet ingredients and mix. Gently stir in the grated zucchini.

Pour mixture into baking pan, and bake for 25-30 minutes, check with a toothpick for doneness.

Let cool before serving.

Vegan Chocolate Cheesecake

Ingredients

Crust
1 cup hazelnut meal
¼ cup + 2 Tablespoons raw cocoa powder
3 Tablespoons maple syrup
1 teaspoon vanilla extract
1 pinch sea salt

Filling

2 cups raw cashews, soaked and rinsed

¼ cup + 2 Tablespoons peanut butter

½ cup coconut oil, melted

½ cup maple syrup

½ cup cocoa powder

½ cup water

½ teaspoon salt

Chocolate Sauce

⅓ cup coconut oil, melted

1 teaspoon vanilla

¼ cup maple syrup

¼ cup cocoa powder

Directions

Blend all crust ingredients together in a food processor until well combined. Press the crust into the bottom of desired pan, about ¼ inch thick and set aside.

In a food processor or mixer blend together cashews, maple syrup, water and salt and mix until smooth, scraping down the sides of the processor if necessary.

Add cocoa powder, hazelnut butter and coconut oil to the cashew mixture and blend together, until mixture is uniformly combined.

Spoon the filling on top of the crust. Place the cheesecake in the freezer for 2 hours or until frozen all the way through.

Once frozen, remove the cheesecake from the pan and place in fridge for 1 hour before serving.

Mix together ingredients for chocolate sauce in a bowl, and drizzle on cake.

Part 2

Introduction

Many people (and even some vegans) do not know that you can make delicious vegan desserts that taste just as good as their non vegan counterparts. This vegan cookbook contains only the best handpicked dairy free vegan baking recipes for you to enjoy!

Chapter 1: Vegan Cake Recipes

Pineapple Upside Down Cake

Ingredients

1.5 cup white flour

1 cup granulated sugar

1 tsp baking soda

1/2 tsp salt

2 1/4 cup Pineapple, canned (reserve juice for use in cake batter)

1/3 cup applesauce, unsweetened

2 tsp lemon juice

1/4 cup brown sugar

2 tsp vanilla extract

Directions

Preheat oven to 350 and spray a baking pan.

Arrange pineapple slices in the pan and set aside.

Mix up the cake batter with everything else except the brown sugar.

Do not over-mix, quickly stir the batter up and pour the batter carefully over the slices. Bake for 25-35 minutes or until done.

Let rest in the pan for a few minutes then flip the cake onto a plate and sprinkle the brown sugar on while it's still very hot.

Let the cake cool for at least 15-20 minutes, and serve.

Banana Chocolate Cake

Ingredients

2 very ripe medium bananas

1 1/4 cups all-purpose (white, unbleached) flour

3/4 cup sugar

1/4 cup unsweetened cocoa powder

1/3 cup canola oil

1/3 cup water

1 teaspoon baking soda

1 teaspoon white vinegar

1/4 teaspoon salt

1/3 cup semisweet vegan chocolate chips

Directions

Preheat oven to 350F.

Mash bananas or blend with electric beater. Blend in wet ingredients and brown sugar.

Sift dry ingredients together then add to wet.

Blend well then pour into 8X8 square cake pan.

Sprinkle chocolate chips over batter.

Bake about 35 minutes or until toothpick inserted in the center comes out clean. Cool completely, about 45 minutes.

Chocolate Vegan Cake

Ingredients

2 cup xylitol

1 3/4 cup flour

3/4 cup cocoa powder

1 1/2 tsp baking powder

1 1/2 tsp baking soda

1 tsp salt

2 portions egg replacer

1 cup soy milk

1/4 cup Lighter Bake

2 tsp vanilla

1 cup boiling water

Directions

Combine all and beat well until well mixed.

Pour into a well prepared bunt cake pan.

Dust with powdered sugar substitute.

Bake at 325F for for 1 hour or until tooth pick inserted in center comes out clean.

Spiced Coconut Cake

Ingredients

1.5 cups of all purpose flour

1 cup sugar

1/2 cup unsweetened coconut

2 tsp cinnamon

1 tsp baking soda

1/4 tsp cayenne pepper

1/4 tsp salt

1 cup cold water

1/4 cup canola oil

1 tbsp balsamic vinegar

1 tablespoon vanilla extract

Directions

Preheat your oven to 350 F

Line the bottom of 10" square cake pan with parchment, and coat sides with cooking spray

Combine all of the cake ingredients in a mixing bowl and stir until smooth

Pour batter into pan and bake 25-30 minutes until toothpick comes out clean. Let cool in pan for 10 minutes

Remove from pan and cool completely.

Vegan Fudge Cake

Ingredients

1 ½ cups sugar

½ cup cocoa

1 ½ teaspoons baking soda

2 cups flour

¾ teaspoon salt

1 ½ teaspoons vanilla

¾ cup vegetable oil

1 ½ cups water

1 ½ teaspoons vinegar

Directions

Preheat oven to 350 degrees.

In an ungreased 9 x 13 pan, sift all dry ingredients.

Add the liquids and stir just until blended. Bake for 25 minutes.

Frost with your choice of frosting.

Vegan Pumpkin Cheesecake

Ingredients

Crust :

2 cups walnuts

1/4 cup maple syrup

4 medjool dates (soaked overnight)

1/2 cup shredded unsweetened coconut

1/4 tsp salt

Filling:

2 cups cashews (soaked min. 4 hours)

1 can pumpkin

6 tbsp coconut oil, melted

3 tbsp. lemon juice

1/4 cup maple syrup

1/2 cup eggnog flavored coconut milk

1/2 cup unsweetened applesauce

1 tsp vanilla extract

2 tsp cinnamon

1/2 tsp nutmeg

1 tsp ground fresh ginger

Directions

Crust :

In food processor, blend dates and maple syrup until smooth, add remaining ingredients pulsing until fully incorporated but still rough texture. Press into 9 inch pie pan

Filling:

In high speed blender, blend all ingredients until smooth and creamy. Pour into crust and freeze for 1-2 hours until firm, not frozen. Defrost 15-20 min. before serving.

Chocolate Zucchini Cake

Ingredients

2 cups grated zucchini

2 tsp vanilla

2 cups whole wheat or whole grain flour

1 tsp salt

1/2 cup light olive oil

1 and 1/4 cup maple syrup

1/4 cup cocoa

1/4 tsp baking soda

Directions

Preheat oven to 350 degrees. Whisk together the dry ingredients.

Add the wet ingredients and mix. Gently stir in the grated zucchini.

Pour into a greased and floured 9 x 13 inch pan, and bake for 25-30 minutes, testing with a toothpick. Remove from oven and let cool before cutting.

Pound Cake

Ingredients

1/2 cup vegan butter, softened

1 1/2 cups granulated or raw sugar

6 ounces plain or low fat Silken firm tofu

2 cups unbleached cake flour

1/2 cups water

2 teaspoons vanilla extract

1 teaspoon almond extract

2 teaspoons baking powder

Directions

Preheat oven to 350 degrees. Lightly grease a 5 x 9" loaf pan. Cream together butter and sugar with an electric mixer on medium speed until fluffy.

Beat in tofu until well combined. Add 1 cup flour and, with mixer on low, mix just until incorporated.

Add water and extracts and do the same. End with remaining cup of flour and baking powder.

Increase speed to medium and beat for 1-2 minutes. Spoon mixture into pan and lightly smooth the top.

Place on the center rack of the oven and bake for 55 minutes.

Orange Cake

Ingredients

1 large orange, peeled

1 1/2 cups all-purpose flour

1 cup white sugar

1/2 cup vegetable oil

1 1/2 teaspoons baking soda

1/4 teaspoon salt

Directions

Preheat oven to 375 degrees F (190 degrees C). Grease an 8x8-inch baking pan.

Blend orange in the blender until liquified; measure 1 cup orange juice.

Whisk orange juice, flour, sugar, vegetable oil, baking soda, and salt together in a bowl. Pour batter into the prepared pan.

Bake in the preheated oven until a toothpick inserted in the center of the cake comes out clean, about 30 minutes.

Creamy Tofu Chocolate Cake

Ingredients

3/4 cup all-purpose flour

1 1/4 cups ground almonds

3/4 cup packed brown sugar, divided

1/2 cup vegan butter

1 1/2 pounds tofu

2/3 cup vegetable oil

1/2 cup orange juice

1/2 cup chocolate liqueur

1/2 cup unsweetened cocoa powder

1 teaspoon almond extract

Directions

Preheat the oven to 325 degrees F (165 degrees C). Lightly grease a 9 inch springform pan.

In a medium bowl, mix together the flour, ground almonds and 1 tablespoon of the brown sugar. Knead in the butter to form a dough. Press the dough firmly into the bottom of the prepared pan.

Using a blender, combine the tofu, remaining sugar, oil, orange juice, chocolate liqueur, cocoa, and almond extract. Blend until smooth and creamy. Spread the batter in an even layer over the prepared crust.

Bake for 1 hour and 15 minutes in the preheated oven. Allow cake to cool to room temperature, then refrigerate overnight.

Chapter 2: Vegan Cookie Recipes

Snickerdoodle Cookies

Ingredients

1 1/2 cups whole wheat flour

1/2 cup white sugar

1/2 teaspoon baking soda

1/2 teaspoon salt

1/2 cup vegetable oil

1 (4 ounce) container applesauce

1 tablespoon vanilla-flavored almond milk

1 tablespoon vanilla extract

1/2 cup cinnamon-sugar

Directions

Preheat oven to 375 degrees F (190 degrees C).

Mix flour, sugar, baking soda, and salt together in a bowl.

Beat vegetable oil, applesauce, almond milk, and vanilla extract together in a separate large bowl; add flour mixture and stir until combined.

Divide dough into 14 portions and roll into balls. Spread cinnamon-sugar into a wide, shallow bowl. Roll dough balls in the cinnamon-sugar and arrange onto a baking sheet.

Bake in preheated oven until golden brown, about 10 minutes.

Gingersnap Cookies

Ingredients

4 tablespoons coarse sugar

2 cups flour

1 teaspoon baking soda

¼ teaspoon salt

2 ½ tablespoons ground ginger

½ teaspoon ground cinnamon

½ teaspoon ground cloves

½ cup canola oil

¼ cup molasses

¼ cup soymilk

1 cup sugar

1 teaspoon vanilla

Directions

Sift dry ingredient (except sugar) into a bowl and set aside.

In a large bowl combine wet ingredients, including sugar and whisk or beat on medium until blended.

Stir in the pre-sifted dry ingredients and mix until well combined.

The dough will be quite sticky and you may need to dampen your hands to work with it. Roll the dough into little balls (about 1 Tablespoon) and flatten out to your liking.

The thinner the cookie the crisper it will be - a slightly thicker cookie will yield a crunch on the edges and a slightly chewy interior.

Press the coarse sugar onto the tops of the cookies and bake about 10 minutes at 350 on a greased cookie sheet.

Vegan Oatmeal Cookies

Ingredients

1 cup white sugar

1/3 cup soy milk

1/3 cup peanut butter

2 tablespoons canola oil

1 teaspoon pure vanilla extract

1 cup whole wheat flour

1 cup rolled oats

1/2 teaspoon baking soda

1/2 teaspoon salt

1/2 cup vegan semi-sweet chocolate chips

1/2 cup walnut pieces

Directions

Preheat oven to 425 degrees F (220 degrees C). Oil a large baking sheet.

Stir sugar, soy milk, peanut butter, canola oil, and vanilla extract together with a whisk in a large bowl until completely smooth.

Mix flour, oats, baking soda, and salt in a separate bowl; add to the peanut butter mixture and stir to combine. Fold chocolate chips and walnut pieces into the flour mixture.

Drop your batter by large spoonfuls onto prepared baking sheet.

Bake cookies in preheated oven until browned along the edges, about 10 minutes. Cool cookies on sheet for 10 minutes before removing to a cooling rack to cool completely.

Chia Seed Cookies

Ingredients

2 cups rolled oats

1 cup brown sugar

2/3 cup whole wheat flour

2 tablespoons chia seeds

1 teaspoon ground cinnamon

1 teaspoon baking soda

1/2 teaspoon baking powder

1/2 teaspoon salt

2/3 cup applesauce

3 tablespoons coconut oil

1 cup dried cranberries

1/2 cup vegan chocolate chips

1/4 cup shredded unsweetened coconut

Directions

Preheat oven to 350 degrees F (175 degrees C). Line a baking sheet with parchment paper.

Combine oats, brown sugar, flour, chia seeds, cinnamon, baking soda, baking powder, and salt in a bowl. Stir applesauce and coconut oil into oat mixture until dough is evenly mixed. Fold cranberries, chocolate chips, and coconut into dough.

Spoon dough onto the prepared baking sheet.

Bake in the preheated oven until edges of cookies are lightly browned, 10 to 15 minutes.

Moist Lemon Cookies

Ingredients

2 ½ cups flour

1 ½ cups sugar

2 teaspoons baking soda

¼ teaspoon salt

2 tablespoons lemon zest

¾ cup canola oil

½ cup lemon juice

2 teaspoons vanilla

Directions

In a medium bowl, stir together flour, sugar, soda, salt, and zest. Make a well in the center and fill with liquid ingredients.

Stir together until well blended. Drop by teaspoonfuls about 2 inches apart on a cookie sheet.

Bake for 8-10 minutes at 350 degrees F.

Chocolate Oatmeal Cookies

Ingredients

2/3 cup maple syrup

1/4 cup vegetable oil

5 tablespoons unsweetened cocoa powder

1 teaspoon ground cinnamon

1/2 cup peanut butter

1 cup rolled oats

1 teaspoon vanilla extract

Directions

In a saucepan over medium heat combine the maple syrup, oil, cocoa and cinnamon. Boil for three minutes, stirring constantly.

Remove from heat and stir in the peanut butter, rolled oats and vanilla until well blended.

Drop by heaping spoonfuls onto waxed paper and chill to set, about 30 minutes.

Banana Oatmeal Cookies

Ingredients

3 large ripe bananas, mashed

2 cups rolled oats

1 cup chopped dates

2 tablespoons applesauce

1 tablespoon vegetable oil

1 teaspoon vanilla extract

2 tablespoons natural peanut butter

1/2 cup vegan chocolate chips

1 teaspoon raw sugar

Directions

Preheat oven to 375 degrees F (190 degrees C). Line a baking sheet with waxed paper.

Mix bananas, oats, dates, applesauce, vegetable oil, and vanilla extract together in a bowl with your hands. Stir in peanut butter until blended; mix in chocolate chips. Let dough stand until oats soften slightly, about 10 minutes.

Drop 1-inch scoops of dough 2 inches apart onto the prepared baking sheet; flatten lightly. Sprinkle raw sugar on top.

Bake in the preheated oven until bottoms are golden, 10 to 15 minutes.

Vegan Butter Cookies

Ingredients

1 cup almond butter

1 cup packed brown sugar

2/3 cup shortening

1/3 cup vegan margarine

1 overripe banana, mashed

2 1/2 cups all-purpose flour

1 1/2 teaspoons baking soda

1 teaspoon baking powder

1/2 teaspoon salt

1 tablespoon water, or as needed

3 ounces vegan dark chocolate, chopped

1/2 cup white sugar

36 whole blanched almonds

Directions

Preheat oven to 375 degrees F (190 degrees C).

Mix almond butter, brown sugar, shortening, and margarine together in a bowl until creamy. Stir in mashed banana.

Combine flour, baking soda, baking powder, and salt in a bowl. Stir into almond butter mixture. Stir in water if dough appears too thick. Fold in dark chocolate.

Pour white sugar onto a shallow dish. Form dough into 1-inch balls and roll in sugar. Arrange 2 inches apart on baking sheets; flatten with a fork. Top each cookie with an almond.

Bake in the preheated oven until lightly browned, about 10 minutes. Cool on the baking sheets for 5 minutes before transferring to a wire rack to cool completely.

Sugar Cookies

Ingredients

1 1/2 cups confectioners' sugar

1 cup vegan margarine

1 1/2 teaspoons vanilla extract

2 1/2 cups all-purpose flour

2 tablespoons cornstarch

1 tablespoon baking powder

1 teaspoon baking soda

all-purpose flour for dusting

Directions

Beat confectioners' sugar and margarine together in a bowl using an electric mixer until smooth and creamy. Add vanilla extract and beat until smooth.

Whisk 2 1/2 cups flour, cornstarch, baking powder, and baking soda together in a separate bowl. Beat flour mixture into creamed butter mixture on medium-low speed just until dough is combined. Separate dough into 2 balls and refrigerate for at least 2 hours.

Preheat oven to 350 degrees F (175 degrees C).

Dust dough with flour and roll into 1/4-inch thick pieces on a work surface. Cut cookies into desired shapes using cookie cutters and arrange on a baking sheet.

Bake in the preheated oven until cookies are just beginning to turn brown, 10 to 14 minutes. Let cookies rest on baking sheet,

5 to 10 minutes; transfer to a wire rack to cool.

Chocolate Fudge Cookies

Ingredients

1 cup whole wheat flour

1/4 teaspoon baking soda

1/8 teaspoon salt

2/3 cup white sugar

7 tablespoons unsweetened cocoa powder

1/3 cup brown sugar

1/3 cup mashed banana

5 tablespoons coconut oil

Directions

Preheat oven to 350 degrees F (175 degrees C).

Mix flour, baking soda, and salt together in a bowl. Combine white sugar, cocoa powder, brown sugar, mashed banana, and coconut together in a saucepan over low heat. Cook and stir until blended and smooth, about 5 minutes. Add flour mixture; stir until smooth dough forms. Drop spoonfuls of dough 2 inches apart onto baking sheets.

Bake in the preheated oven until edges are golden, about 8 minutes.

Peanut Butter Cookies

Ingredients

1/2 Cup agave nectar

1/4 cup brown rice syrup

1/3 cup grapeseed oil

2/3 cup peanut butter

2 tablespoons almond milk

1 tablespoon ground flax seeds

2 teaspoons pure vanilla extract

1/4 teaspoon almond extract

1 1/2 cup all purpose flour

3/4 cup whole wheat flour

1 teaspoon baking soda

1/4 teaspoon salt

Directions

Preheat oven to 325F.

Whisk together agave nectar, syrup, oil, peanut butter, nondairy milk, flax seeds, and extract until smooth. Sift in the flour, baking soda, salt, and mix.

Drop on sheet, bake for 12 to 14 minutes.

Chapter 3: Vegan Muffin Recipes

Banana Muffins

Ingredients

3 cups all-purpose flour

1 cup white sugar

1/2 cup brown sugar

2 teaspoons ground cinnamon

2 teaspoons baking powder

1 teaspoon baking soda

1 teaspoon ground nutmeg

1 teaspoon salt

2 cups mashed ripe bananas

1 cup canola oil

1 cup coconut milk

Directions

Preheat oven to 350 degrees F (175 degrees C). Grease 12 muffin cups or line with paper liners.

Mix flour, white sugar, brown sugar, cinnamon, baking powder, baking soda, nutmeg, and salt together in a large bowl. Stir bananas, canola oil, and coconut milk together in a separate bowl; mix banana mixture into flour mixture until just combined. Fill muffin cups with batter.

Bake in the preheated oven until a tooth pick inserted in the center of a muffin comes out clean, 30 to 35 minutes.

Oat Muffins

Ingredients

3 cups oat flour

5 tablespoons raw sunflower seeds

3 tablespoons raw pumpkin seeds

- 1 tablespoon baking powder
- 1 1/2 teaspoons ground cinnamon
- 1/2 teaspoon ground nutmeg
- 1/2 teaspoon ground ginger
- 1/2 teaspoon salt
- 1/4 teaspoon ground cloves
- 3 tablespoons hot water
- 1 tablespoon flax seed meal
- 1 1/4 cups soy milk
- 1/2 cup raisins
- 6 tablespoons agave nectar, or more to taste
- 1 1/2 tablespoons olive oil

Directions

Preheat oven to 350 degrees F (175 degrees C). Grease 12 muffin cups or spray with cooking spray.

Mix oat flour, sunflower seeds, pumpkin seeds, baking powder, cinnamon, nutmeg, ginger, salt, and cloves together in a bowl.

Stir hot water and flax seed meal together in a small bowl; add to flour mixture. Stir soy milk, raisins, agave nectar, and olive oil into flour mixture until batter is just mixed.

Scoop batter into the prepared muffin cups using an ice cream scoop.

Bake in the preheated oven until a toothpick inserted in the center of a muffin comes out clean, 25 to 30 minutes.

Cornbread Muffins

Ingredients

1/2 cup cornmeal

1/2 cup whole-wheat pastry flour

1/2 teaspoon baking soda

1/2 teaspoon salt

1/2 cup applesauce

1/2 cup soy milk

1/4 cup agave nectar

2 tablespoons canola oil

Directions

Preheat oven to 325 degrees F (165 degrees C). Lightly grease a muffin pan.

Combine the cornmeal, flour, baking soda, and salt in a large bowl; stir in the applesauce, soy milk, and agave nectar. Slowly add the oil while stirring. Pour the mixture into the muffin pan.

Bake in the preheated oven until a toothpick or small knife inserted in the crown of a muffin comes out clean, 15 to 20 minutes.

Apple Carrot Muffins

Ingredients

1 cup brown sugar

1/2 cup white sugar

2 1/2 cups all-purpose flour

4 teaspoons baking soda

1 teaspoon baking powder

4 teaspoons ground cinnamon

2 teaspoons salt

2 cups finely grated carrots

2 large apples - peeled, cored and shredded

6 teaspoons egg replacer (dry)

1 1/4 cups applesauce

1/4 cup vegetable oil

Directions

Preheat oven to 375 degrees F (190 degrees C). Grease muffin cups or line with paper muffin liners.

In a large bowl combine brown sugar, white sugar, flour, baking soda, baking powder, cinnamon and salt. Stir in carrot and apple; mix well.

In a small bowl whisk together egg substitute, applesauce and oil. Stir into dry ingredients.

Spoon batter into prepared pans.

Bake in preheated oven for 20 minutes. Let muffins cool in pan for 5 minutes before removing from pans to cool completely.

Pumpkin Muffins

Ingredients

2 cups whole wheat flour

1/2 cup packed brown sugar

1 tablespoon baking powder

1 teaspoon ground cinnamon

1/2 teaspoon baking soda

1/2 teaspoon salt

1/2 teaspoon ground nutmeg

1 (15 ounce) can solid-pack pumpkin

1/2 cup water

1/2 cup vegan chocolate chips

Directions

Preheat oven to 375 degrees F (190 degrees C). Line 12 muffin cups with paper liners.

Whisk whole wheat flour, brown sugar, baking powder, cinnamon, baking soda, salt, and nutmeg in a large bowl. Stir pumpkin and water into dry ingredients, mixing until just moistened; fold in chocolate chips.

Spoon batter into prepared muffin cups, filling them to just below the tops.

Bake in the preheated oven until lightly browned and tops of muffins bounce back when pressed lightly, 25 to 30 minutes.

Let muffins cool in pans for 5 minutes until removing to a wire rack to cool completely.

Classic Zucchini Muffins

Ingredients

1/4 cup chia seeds

1 cup water

1 cup cashew flour

- 1/4 cup ground flax seed
- 2 tablespoons coconut flour
- 2 tablespoons tapioca starch
- 1 tablespoon ground cinnamon
- 1 teaspoon baking soda
- 1/2 teaspoon salt
- 1 cup chopped dates
- 1 cup chopped walnuts
- 1 cup shredded zucchini
- 1/3 cup applesauce
- 2 tablespoons coconut oil, melted
- 1 fluid ounce liquid stevia, or to taste

Directions

Preheat oven to 375 degrees F (190 degrees C). Line 12 muffin cups with paper liners.

Soak chia seeds in the water in a bowl until thickened and paste-like, 5 to 10 minutes.

Whisk cashew flour, flax seed, coconut flour, tapioca starch, cinnamon, baking soda, and salt together in a bowl.

Mix chia seed mixture, dates, walnuts, zucchini, applesauce, coconut oil, and stevia together in a separate bowl; stir into dry mixture until batter is just combined. Spoon batter into the muffin cups.

Bake in the preheated oven until a toothpick inserted in the middle of a muffin comes out clean, 30 to 35 minutes.

Cool muffins in the muffin tin on a wire rack before removing, about 10 minutes; cool another 5 minutes before serving.

Pecan Muffins

Ingredients

9 tablespoons water

- 3 tablespoons flax seed meal
- 1 1/4 cups gluten-free all-purpose flour
- 3 tablespoons chopped pecans
- 2 tablespoons coconut flour
- 1 teaspoon baking soda
- 1 teaspoon baking powder
- 1/4 teaspoon salt
- 1/2 cup maple syrup
- 3 tablespoons coconut oil
- 1 teaspoon vanilla extract

Directions

Preheat oven to 350 degrees F (175 degrees C). Grease 9 muffin cups or line with paper liners.

Stir water and flax seed meal together in a bowl; set aside until "flax egg" is thickened, about 10 minutes.

Whisk gluten-free all-purpose flour, pecans, coconut flour, baking soda, baking powder, and salt together in a large bowl. Add flax egg, maple syrup, coconut oil, and vanilla extract to flour mixture and mix well until batter is smooth.

Scoop batter into the prepared muffin cups.

Bake in the preheated oven until muffin tops are starting to brown, about 17 minutes.

Cool muffins in the tin for a few minutes before removing.

Bran Muffins

Ingredients

1 1/4 cups bran flakes cereal

1 1/4 cups all-purpose flour

1/3 cup brown sugar

1 teaspoon ground cinnamon

1 tablespoon baking powder

1 1/4 cups apple juice

1/4 cup margarine, melted

1 teaspoon vanilla extract

1 apple - peeled, cored and chopped

Directions

Preheat oven to 375 degrees F (190 degrees C). Grease muffin tins.

In a mixing bowl, combine bran flakes, flour, brown sugar, cinnamon and baking powder. Stir in apple juice, margarine, vanilla, and apple. Spoon the mixture into the greased muffin tins.

Bake at 375 degrees F (190 degrees C) for 25 to 30 minutes.

About the Author

Jessie Mills is author of several cookbooks on Vegan diet. He has written research papers on the topic and currently lives in California.

www.ingramcontent.com/pod-product-compliance
Lightning Source LLC
LaVergne TN
LVHW012000070526
838202LV00054B/4976